Biologics and Skin Health

Understanding Biologics with Aesthetic Therapies

Amy Jo Roberts, LE

To all the estheticians who dream of doing more with their license, this book is for you. I see your passion, your curiosity, and your drive to go beyond the treatment room. You are the future of this industry. Never stop digging deeper into your craft and exploring what truly excites you. Dive into the research, yes, even PubMed. The studies and science are there for us, too. They hold the keys to understanding how ingredients and biologics interact with the skin on a cellular level.

Continue to challenge yourself to grow. Learn, experiment, and master the art of connecting science with hands-on care. Remember, the doctors need us as collaborators, educators, and partners in advancing skin health.

And most importantly—have fun. Stay inspired. Keep your love for this work alive. You are changing lives, one client at a time, and your journey has only just begun.

-Amy

Copyright Page

This publication is designed to provide accurate and authoritative information in regard to the subject matter covered. It is provided with the understanding that neither the author nor the publisher is engaged in rendering legal, medical, investment, accounting, or other professional services. If professional advice or assistance is required, the services of a qualified professional should be sought.

While every effort has been made to ensure the accuracy and completeness of the information contained in this book, the author and publisher make no representations or warranties, express or implied, regarding its accuracy, reliability, or completeness. They specifically disclaim any implied warranties of merchantability or fitness for a particular purpose. No warranty may be created or extended by any promotional statements or materials.

The advice and strategies contained herein may not be suitable for every individual or situation. The reader assumes full responsibility for how the information is used. Neither the author nor the publisher shall be liable for any loss of profit, personal injury, or any other damages, including but not limited to incidental, consequential, or other damages arising from the use or misuse of this material.

This book is intended for educational and informational purposes only, particularly within the field of esthetics, skin health, and regenerative aesthetics. It is not intended to diagnose, treat, cure, or prevent any medical condition. Readers should consult with a licensed healthcare provider or qualified professional before making any decisions related to medical treatments or procedures.

References to biologics, including but not limited to exosomes, peptides, purified amniotic fluid, and related materials, are provided for educational context only. These substances may be subject to regulatory oversight and varying legal status depending on jurisdiction. This publication does not promote or imply use outside of approved indications or scope of practice.

Individual results may vary. The author makes no guarantees regarding outcomes.

First Edition 2025

Overview

Biologics and Skin Health is a groundbreaking guide that bridges the worlds of aesthetic science and regenerative medicine. Written for estheticians, medical professionals, and skin health enthusiasts, this book explores the transformative power of biologically active ingredients in modern skincare.

From Purified Amniotic Fluid to Wharton's Jelly and exosomes, Amy Roberts, LE, demystifies these advanced therapies with clear, science-backed explanations and practical protocols. Drawing on over 10 years of hands-on experience as a Licensed Esthetician in two states—and her collaboration with a regenerative medicine scientist—Amy provides readers with unique insights into how biologics work at the cellular level to promote repair, regeneration, and rejuvenation.

This comprehensive resource not only unpacks the science behind these bioactive molecules but also equips readers with actionable knowledge for integrating biologics into professional practice. With chapters covering skin structure and wound healing, treatment pairings, post-care optimization, and ethical considerations, this book serves as both a scientific reference and a practical training manual.

Whether you are an experienced practitioner seeking to elevate your treatments or a newcomer to the field of aesthetics, **Biologics and Skin Health** offers the tools, confidence, and expertise to embrace the next generation of skin rejuvenation.

Table of Contents

Chapter 1

Introduction to Biologics

What Are Biologics?

Biologics are advanced therapeutic products derived from living organisms. They are used in medicine and aesthetics to promote healing, regenerate tissue, reduce inflammation, and enhance overall skin function. Unlike traditional synthetic drugs, biologics are complex and bioactive, meaning they interact directly with the body's cellular systems.

Key Characteristics of Biologics

Biologics are therapeutic agents derived from living cells or tissues, including human, animal, or microbial sources. Unlike traditional pharmaceuticals that are chemically synthesized, biologics are complex in structure and exhibit biological activity at a cellular level. This complexity allows them to interact with the body more dynamically, often mimicking or enhancing natural cellular processes. In aesthetics, biologics are typically administered through injection, topical application, or microneedling to penetrate the dermal layers effectively. Their ability to engage with skin cells, stimulate repair pathways, and modulate inflammatory responses makes them a cornerstone of regenerative treatments.

Types of Biologics Used in Aesthetic Treatments

Several types of biologics have become prominent in the field of aesthetics:

1. Platelet-Rich Plasma (PRP): An autologous therapy created from the patient's own blood, PRP is rich in growth factors that accelerate wound healing and stimulate collagen production. It has gained popularity for its use in facial rejuvenation and hair restoration.

2. Purified Amniotic Fluid (PAF): Sourced from donated placental tissue, PAF is a potent anti-inflammatory and regenerative fluid. It contains a rich array of exosomes, growth factors, cytokines, and lipids, which support skin healing and enhance post-procedural recovery. I like to refer to it as the full orchestra of biologics.

3. Wharton's Jelly: Harvested from the umbilical cord matrix, Wharton's Jelly is abundant in mesenchymal signaling molecules and extracellular matrix components. These extracts are used to promote

advanced skin regeneration and are increasingly favored for their role in scar revision and anti-aging treatments.

4. Exosomes: These nanovesicles carry proteins, lipids, and RNA, serving as messengers to stimulate cellular repair and regeneration. Exosomes are emerging as a powerful addition to microneedling and laser treatments for their ability to activate cellular communication pathways.

There are also products on the market that have been lyophilized, or freeze-dried, and are often grouped into the biologics category. However, it is important to understand that these are not the same as preserved, intact biologic systems. To lyophilize a product, the original cellular structure is no longer maintained in the same way, which changes how the skin can interpret and respond to it. Because of this, these products are not always recognized by the skin as a true signaling system. In many cases, the primary functional component that remains active is the hyaluronic acid, providing hydration but not the same level of coordinated communication. While they may still offer some surface-level benefits, they do not replicate the integrated, multi-signal environment of a complete biologic, and their results tend to be more limited in comparison.

How Biologics Benefit the Skin

The application of biologics in aesthetics has shown profound effects on skin health and appearance. They promote the production of collagen and elastin, two essential proteins that provide skin its structure and elasticity. By enhancing wound healing and reducing inflammation, biologics help repair damaged tissue and soothe irritated skin. Clinically, they improve overall skin texture, tone, and pigmentation irregularities. Furthermore, their regenerative properties help reduce visible signs of aging, including fine lines and wrinkles, while supporting increased cellular turnover for a refreshed and youthful glow.

Common Aesthetic Applications

Biologics have found versatile applications across aesthetic procedures:

<u>Microneedling with PRP or Purified Amniotic Fluid</u>: These combinations amplify the benefits of microneedling by delivering growth factors directly into the microchannels created during treatment. When utilizing PRP, the growth

factors are only as good as the patient, while purified amniotic fluid presents the best quality of growth factors and brings along exosomes, Klotho, and all the other proteins benefiting regeneration.

Post-Laser and RF Microneedling Recovery: Biologic serums applied post-procedure enhance healing, reduce downtime, and improve outcomes.

Topical Use in Anti-Aging Facials: As part of luxury facials, biologics can elevate results by infusing skin with regenerative molecules.

Hair Restoration Protocols: PRP, PAF, Wharton's Jelly, and Exosomes are frequently used in scalp treatments to stimulate hair follicle activity and promote new hair growth.

Acne Scar Repair: Biologics assist in remodeling scar tissue and restoring smoother skin texture.

Legal and Regulatory Considerations

Estheticians should always operate within their professional licensing regulations, scope of practice, and applicable state guidelines when incorporating biologic-based ingredients into aesthetic treatments. In many aesthetic settings, biologic ingredients are intended for topical cosmetic application and skin-supportive care rather than medical treatment.

Regulatory oversight may vary depending on factors such as formulation, processing methods, sourcing, marketing claims, and intended use. Because the biologics landscape continues to evolve, professionals need to prioritize education, compliance, and responsible product integration. Practitioners should also verify that products are sourced from reputable, compliant manufacturers and tissue banks when applicable.

Many biologic ingredients discussed within aesthetics are manufactured and marketed for topical cosmetic use. Professionals should always follow manufacturer guidelines and avoid applications that fall outside their licensing or intended product use.

Biologics represent an emerging frontier within regenerative aesthetics and advanced skincare education. When integrated appropriately within professional scope and cosmetic application guidelines, these ingredients may help support skin recovery, post-treatment care, overall skin appearance, and treatment outcomes. Continued education, ethical practice, and regulatory awareness remain essential as biologic technologies continue to evolve within the aesthetic industry.

Chapter 2

The Science of Skin Regeneration

Skin Structure and the Wound Healing Cascade

The human skin is the largest organ of the body, serving as a complex barrier that protects internal tissues from environmental stressors, pathogens, and mechanical injury. It is composed of three primary layers, each with distinct structural and functional roles essential for maintaining homeostasis and supporting regeneration after injury.

Layers of the Skin

Epidermis: The outermost layer, primarily made of keratinocytes, acts as a protective shield against physical, chemical, and microbial assaults. It undergoes constant renewal through basal cell proliferation and migration toward the surface, where cells are eventually shed.

Dermis: Situated beneath the epidermis, the dermis consists of collagen, elastin, and an extracellular matrix (ECM) that provide tensile strength and elasticity. This layer houses blood vessels, lymphatics, nerves, hair follicles, and sweat glands, playing a critical role in thermoregulation and sensation.

Subcutaneous Tissue (Hypodermis): The deepest layer, composed mainly of adipose tissue, cushions and insulates the body while serving as an energy reserve. It connects the dermis to underlying muscles and supports the skin's flexibility.

The Wound Healing Cascade

When the skin sustains an injury or controlled micro-trauma, such as during microneedling or laser resurfacing, it activates a highly coordinated process known as the wound healing cascade. This cascade facilitates repair and restoration of skin integrity and consists of four overlapping but distinct phases:

1. Hemostasis (Minutes to Hours):
   Immediately after injury, blood vessels constrict to minimize blood loss, and platelets aggregate to form a clot. This clot acts as a temporary matrix and releases growth factors like platelet-derived growth factor (PDGF) and vascular endothelial growth factor (VEGF) to recruit immune cells and kickstart healing.
2. Inflammation (1–3 Days):
   Neutrophils and macrophages infiltrate the wound site to remove pathogens, dead cells, and debris. These immune cells release cytokines and

chemokines, creating a pro-inflammatory environment that signals fibroblasts and keratinocytes to begin repair. Mild erythema and swelling, often observed after aesthetic treatments, are hallmarks of this phase.

3. Proliferation (4–21 Days):
   Fibroblasts and keratinocytes are the key players in this stage. Fibroblasts synthesize new collagen and ECM proteins, while keratinocytes migrate from the wound edges to cover the injury. Angiogenesis occurs, forming new blood vessels to supply nutrients and oxygen to regenerating tissues. Clinically, this is when visible improvements in skin texture and tone often begin to emerge.
4. Remodeling (21 Days to 1 Year):
   Collagen fibers mature and reorganize into a stronger, more structured matrix. Type III collagen initially laid down during proliferation is replaced by Type I collagen, restoring the skin's tensile strength. Over time, the vascularity of the area diminishes, and the repaired tissue blends with the surrounding skin.

Aesthetic Relevance

Controlled micro-injury, as induced by microneedling, laser, or radiofrequency treatments, strategically triggers this cascade to remodel and rejuvenate skin. Pairing these techniques with biologics, such as platelet-rich plasma (PRP), purified amniotic fluid, or exosomes, introduces additional growth factors and cytokines that can accelerate and enhance each phase of healing. This leads to faster recovery, reduced downtime, and superior aesthetic outcomes.

Role of Fibroblasts, Keratinocytes, and Growth Factors

The skin's remarkable ability to repair and renew itself after injury relies on the orchestrated action of specialized cells and biochemical signals. Among these, fibroblasts, keratinocytes, and growth factors play central roles in both natural wound healing and the mechanisms leveraged in aesthetic treatments. Understanding their functions provides insight into why biologics such as PRP, purified amniotic fluid, and exosomes are so effective in regenerative aesthetics.

Fibroblasts: The Architects of the Dermis

Fibroblasts are the primary cells responsible for rebuilding the dermal matrix. Located within the dermis, they are activated during the proliferation phase of wound healing and are critical for the synthesis of extracellular matrix (ECM) components like collagen and elastin. These structural proteins provide tensile strength and elasticity to the skin.

In regenerative treatments, stimulating fibroblasts accelerates the production of new collagen (particularly Type I and III) and hyaluronic acid, leading to firmer, smoother, and more youthful skin. Biologic agents enhance fibroblast activity, encouraging faster remodeling and scar softening.

Keratinocytes: The Guardians of the Epidermis

Keratinocytes make up about 90% of the epidermal cells and are vital for the re-epithelialization process following skin injury. These cells migrate from the wound edges to cover exposed dermal tissue, restoring the protective barrier of the skin.

Keratinocytes also release cytokines and chemokines during the inflammatory phase, signaling fibroblasts and immune cells to coordinate the healing process. In aesthetic procedures, supporting keratinocyte proliferation is crucial for achieving an even skin tone and preventing post-inflammatory hyperpigmentation.

Growth Factors: The Molecular Messengers

Growth factors are naturally occurring proteins that regulate cellular communication during tissue repair. They act as biochemical signals that stimulate cell proliferation, migration, and differentiation. Key growth factors include:

- Epidermal Growth Factor (EGF): Promotes keratinocyte and fibroblast proliferation, speeding up wound closure and skin rejuvenation.
- Fibroblast Growth Factor (FGF): Encourages angiogenesis (formation of new blood vessels) and stimulates fibroblasts to produce ECM.
- Platelet-Derived Growth Factor (PDGF): Attracts fibroblasts and smooth muscle cells to the wound site, enhancing tissue remodeling.
- Transforming Growth Factor-Beta (TGF-β): Regulates collagen synthesis and modulates the inflammatory response.

Clinical Relevance in Biologic Therapies

Biologic-based treatments leverage these natural cellular mechanisms to accelerate repair and improve aesthetic outcomes. Exosomes and amniotic fluid, for example, are rich in signaling molecules that directly influence fibroblast and keratinocyte behavior, allowing for faster recovery and enhanced collagen remodeling with less downtime.

Cellular Aging and Repair Mechanisms

Aging is a complex biological process that affects every cell and tissue in the human body, including the skin. At the cellular level, aging is marked by cumulative damage and declining repair capacity, leading to visible signs such as wrinkles, thinning, laxity, and uneven pigmentation. Understanding these mechanisms is crucial for developing and applying regenerative aesthetic treatments that target aging at its root.

The Hallmarks of Cellular Aging in Skin

As we age, several key cellular processes begin to falter:

Slowed Cellular Turnover: The basal layer of the epidermis produces new keratinocytes at a slower rate, resulting in dullness and delayed wound healing.

DNA Damage Accumulation: Environmental stressors such as UV radiation, pollution, and toxins lead to DNA mutations. With age, DNA repair pathways become less efficient, allowing damage to accumulate.

Oxidative Stress: Reactive oxygen species (ROS) generated by metabolism and external stress oxidize lipids, proteins, and DNA. Over time, this oxidative damage degrades skin structure.

Telomere Shortening: Each cell division causes progressive loss of telomeres, the protective caps on chromosomes. When telomeres become critically short, cells enter senescence or programmed cell death (apoptosis).

Reduced Growth Factor Signaling: Aging fibroblasts secrete fewer growth factors like EGF and TGF-β, leading to impaired collagen synthesis and slower tissue repair.

Intrinsic Repair Mechanisms

Despite these challenges, the skin has remarkable intrinsic repair systems that can be stimulated through aesthetic interventions:

Mitochondrial Function Enhancement: Healthy mitochondria provide the energy needed for cell renewal. Treatments that stimulate mitochondrial biogenesis can help reverse cellular energy deficits.

Autophagy Activation: Autophagy, literally meaning "self-eating," is a process by which cells remove damaged organelles and proteins. Reactivating autophagy in aging skin promotes detoxification and renewal, making cells more resilient to stress.

Stem Cell Activity: Resident stem cells in the basal epidermis and dermis can differentiate into new keratinocytes and fibroblasts, maintaining skin homeostasis when adequately supported.

Klotho: The Anti-Aging Protein Unique to Purified Amniotic Fluid

A standout discovery in regenerative medicine is Klotho, often referred to as the "longevity protein." Named after the Greek goddess of fate who spins the thread of life, Klotho plays a key role in regulating cellular aging and longevity.

What is Klotho?

Klotho is a transmembrane protein with anti-aging properties. It protects cells from oxidative stress, supports DNA repair, and regulates calcium and phosphate metabolism. Reduced Klotho expression is associated with accelerated aging, skin atrophy, and delayed wound healing.

Why Purified Amniotic Fluid?

Unlike other biologic materials, purified amniotic fluid contains abundant Klotho, offering a unique advantage in aesthetic therapies. Its presence contributes to the unparalleled regenerative potential of purified amniotic fluid (PAF) when applied topically or via microneedling.

Aesthetic Implications:

Treatments using PAF naturally containing Klotho can promote youthful cellular function, enhance mitochondrial efficiency, and counteract oxidative stress. This results in visibly firmer, more radiant skin with reduced signs of aging.

Aesthetic Applications: Reversing Cellular Aging

Modern regenerative aesthetic treatments harness these repair mechanisms to rejuvenate aging skin:

Microneedling & Lasers: Induce controlled micro-trauma, triggering a healing response that reactivates fibroblasts and stimulates collagen and elastin production.

Biologic Agents (PRP, Exosomes, Purified Amniotic Fluid):

Deliver concentrated growth factors and signaling molecules that enhance cellular communication and repair, with purified amniotic fluid offering the added benefit of Klotho.

Energy-Based Devices: Technologies like LED light therapy or acoustic wave devices improve mitochondrial health and circulation, amplifying repair processes.

By addressing cellular aging at multiple levels of energy production, detoxification, and signaling, these therapies restore youthful vitality to the skin.

Chapter 3

Overview of Key Biologic Ingredients

Exosomes: What They Are and How They Signal Skin Repair

Exosomes represent one of the most exciting frontiers in regenerative aesthetics. These nano-sized extracellular vesicles, secreted by virtually all cell types, especially mesenchymal signaling cells, act as critical messengers in the body's cellular communication network. Understanding their function provides key insights into their transformative potential in aesthetic practice.

What Are Exosomes?

Exosomes are lipid bilayer vesicles ranging from 30 to 150 nanometers in diameter. They are formed inside cells and released into the extracellular environment as part of normal physiological processes. Often described as "cellular delivery vehicles," exosomes contain a cargo of bioactive molecules, including:

- Proteins (e.g., growth factors, enzymes)
- Lipids (for membrane structure and signaling)

- mRNA and microRNA (to influence gene expression in recipient cells)

How Do Exosomes Signal Skin Repair?

Exosomes play a pivotal role in skin regeneration by acting as signaling hubs in the wound healing cascade:
Reducing Inflammation: Exosomes carry anti-inflammatory molecules that modulate immune responses, reducing redness and swelling after aesthetic procedures.

Stimulating Fibroblasts: Once absorbed into dermal tissue, exosomes deliver microRNA and proteins that activate fibroblasts, prompting them to synthesize new collagen and elastin.

Promoting Angiogenesis: Exosomal cargo includes vascular endothelial growth factor (VEGF), encouraging the formation of new blood vessels to supply nutrients and oxygen to regenerating skin.

Enhancing Cellular Turnover: By transferring mRNA and regulatory microRNAs, exosomes "reprogram" aging or stressed cells, restoring their youthful function and improving overall skin vitality.

Aesthetic Applications of Exosomes

In clinical practice, exosomes are increasingly used in combination with minimally invasive treatments to amplify results:

Microneedling + Exosomes: Applied immediately post-procedure, exosomes penetrate microchannels to accelerate healing and enhance collagen remodeling.

Laser & RF Treatments: Used topically after ablative procedures, exosomes reduce downtime and improve outcomes by supporting rapid epidermal repair.

Facial Rejuvenation Serums: As a topical therapy, exosomes help maintain skin health by reducing oxidative stress and boosting hydration.

Scar Revision & Hair Restoration: Exosome therapies have shown promise in improving scar texture and stimulating dormant hair follicles.

Why Exosomes Over PRP?

Unlike PRP, which depends on a patient's blood composition, exosomes offer a standardized, cell-free alternative rich in growth factors and signaling molecules. They are hypoallergenic and safe for all skin types, making them an excellent adjunct to aesthetic treatments for diverse patient populations.

Amniotic Fluid: Anti-Inflammatory and Regenerative Properties

In the field of regenerative aesthetics, purified amniotic fluid (PAF) stands out as a multifaceted biologic with unparalleled healing potential. Derived from ethically donated full-term cesarian birth placental tissue and processed to ensure purity and safety, PAF delivers a rich array of bioactive molecules that orchestrate cellular renewal and repair.

What Is Amniotic Fluid?

Amniotic fluid is the protective liquid that surrounds a developing fetus during pregnancy. It provides a nurturing environment rich in growth factors, cytokines, hyaluronic acid, and extracellular vesicles like exosomes. When purified for medical and aesthetic use, this fluid retains its regenerative components while being free of cells and DNA, minimizing any immunogenic response.

This unique biologic acts as a "cell-free therapy," delivering a comprehensive cocktail of molecules that communicate with skin cells to stimulate rejuvenation and healing.

A Symphony of Healing Molecules

Using purified amniotic fluid in aesthetics is akin to having an entire orchestra play in harmony rather than listening to a single instrument.

Instead of relying on one growth factor or cytokine, PAF provides a balanced and synergistic blend of:

1. Growth Factors: Including epidermal growth factor (EGF), transforming growth factor-beta (TGF-β), and vascular endothelial growth factor (VEGF) to drive cell proliferation and angiogenesis.
2. Cytokines: Anti-inflammatory messengers that help modulate immune responses and reduce redness, swelling, and irritation post-treatment.
3. Exosomes: Nano-sized vesicles that carry proteins and RNA to support cellular communication and repair.
4. Hyaluronic Acid: A natural humectant that provides deep hydration, plumping the skin and supporting barrier function.
5. Klotho: A transmembrane protein with anti-aging properties. It protects cells from oxidative stress,

supports DNA repair, and regulates calcium and phosphate metabolism. Reduced Klotho expression is associated with accelerated aging, skin atrophy, and delayed wound healing.

Anti-Inflammatory Benefits

One of PAF's defining attributes is its potent anti-inflammatory effect. By downregulating pro-inflammatory cytokines and upregulating anti-inflammatory mediators, PAF helps soothe irritated skin, reduce erythema, and accelerate the resolution of post-procedure inflammation. This makes it an ideal adjunct to treatments like microneedling, lasers, or chemical peels.

Regenerative and Rejuvenating Effects

Beyond calming the skin, PAF helps support regeneration:

Helps Stimulate Fibroblast Activity: Enhances collagen and elastin synthesis for improved skin firmness and elasticity.

Helps Accelerate Wound Healing: Shortening recovery times and helping to reduce the risk of post-inflammatory pigmentation.

Helps Promote Skin Hydration: Restores moisture balance and supports a healthier, more youthful appearance.

Applications in Aesthetics

Purified Amniotic Fluid has shown versatility in practice:

Microneedling Adjunct: Applied post-treatment, PAF helps speed healing and amplifies collagen remodeling.

Post-Laser Care: Helps soothe the skin and supports re-epithelialization after ablative or fractional laser procedures.

Facial Rejuvenation: Used as part of luxury facials to help hydrate, calm, and repair stressed or aging skin.

Scar and Stretch Mark Treatment: Helps support remodeling of scar tissue for smoother, more uniform skin texture.

Peptides

Messengers in Topical Form

Modern aesthetic science has uncovered the transformative potential of biologically active molecules for skin rejuvenation. At the forefront of this innovation are peptides, short chains of amino acids that act as potent signaling molecules within the skin's intricate cellular network.

Peptides serve as messengers that communicate specific instructions to skin cells, encouraging them to perform essential functions such as repairing damaged tissue, boosting collagen and elastin production, and regulating inflammatory responses. Unlike larger proteins, their small molecular size allows them to penetrate the skin barrier more effectively, making them ideal for topical delivery.

When incorporated into advanced skincare formulations and post-procedure serums, peptides provide a non-invasive yet highly effective pathway to regenerative outcomes. They have been shown to improve skin firmness, reduce the appearance of fine lines and wrinkles, enhance hydration, and support the skin's natural barrier function.

In the context of aesthetics, peptides complement in-office procedures by accelerating recovery and amplifying treatment results. For example, applying peptide-rich serums after microneedling or LED therapy enhances absorption through temporarily opened microchannels, maximizing their bioactivity.

This growing category of bioactive ingredients has made peptides a cornerstone of modern anti-aging and reparative skincare, offering clients both immediate and long-term improvements in skin quality.

What Are Peptides?

Peptides are short chains of amino acids, the building blocks of proteins, linked by peptide bonds. Unlike larger proteins, their small size allows them to penetrate the outer layers of the skin and interact with cellular receptors. Peptides function as signaling molecules, instructing skin cells on how to behave for optimal regeneration.

Key Functions of Peptides in Aesthetic Care:

Stimulate Collagen Production: Certain peptides, such as palmitoyl pentapeptide (Matrixyl), signal fibroblasts to synthesize new collagen, improving skin firmness and reducing fine lines.

Support Barrier Repair: Peptides help restore the skin's lipid barrier, preventing water loss and improving resilience against environmental aggressors.

Control Inflammation: Some peptides possess anti-inflammatory properties that calm irritated skin and reduce redness post-treatment.

Act as Antioxidants: Copper peptides help neutralize free radicals and enhance wound healing by supporting angiogenesis.

Topical Application: How They Work

While peptides naturally exist in the skin, their levels diminish with age. Topical delivery replenishes these critical molecules, acting as a "cellular whisperer" to encourage youthful function. Advanced formulations encapsulate these proteins in liposomes or nanocarriers, ensuring they remain stable and bioactive until they reach target skin layers.

Benefits in Aesthetics

Peptides are key components in post-procedure serums and luxury skincare lines.

Their benefits include:

Faster recovery after microneedling, laser, or RF treatments.

Improved hydration and barrier repair for sensitive skin types.

Reduced inflammation and erythema for clients prone to redness.

Gradual enhancement of skin tone, texture, and elasticity with regular use.

Understanding Water-Based and Oil-Based Peptides

Peptides have become a cornerstone of modern aesthetic science, celebrated for their ability to signal skin cells to repair, rebuild, and rejuvenate. However, the effectiveness of peptides in skincare is not only determined by their molecular composition but also by the formulation base, whether water or oil, and the timing of their application after a procedure. Understanding how these formulations interact with the skin's biology is essential for maximizing their benefits.

Why Start with a Water-Based Peptide?

Peptides are hydrophilic molecules by nature. Their structure, composed of chains of amino acids, is water-soluble, meaning they dissolve readily in aqueous solutions. This property allows peptides in water-based serums to penetrate more efficiently into the skin's upper layers, especially when applied immediately after procedures like microneedling or dermaplaning.

Post-treatment, the skin's barrier is temporarily compromised. Microchannels created during treatments increase permeability, allowing water-soluble peptides to travel to deeper layers of the epidermis where they can activate fibroblasts, stimulate collagen production, and initiate repair processes.

Because of their hydrophilic (water-loving) nature, water-based peptides should always be applied first in a post-treatment regimen. Their small size and compatibility with the skin's aqueous environment enable them to diffuse into the extracellular matrix, where they can bind to receptors and trigger cellular responses.

Transitioning to Oil-Based Peptides for Barrier Repair

Approximately 48 hours after treatment, as the skin's natural barrier begins to recover, oil-based peptides can be introduced. These formulations typically feature lipophilic (oil-loving) peptide derivatives or encapsulations that allow them to function differently than their water-based counterparts.

Lipophilic molecules are attracted to lipids and can integrate into the lipid-rich environment of the stratum corneum (the outermost layer of the skin). This makes them ideal for barrier support. By applying oil-based peptides at this stage, they act as an occlusive layer, preventing trans epidermal water loss (TEWL), enhancing hydration retention, and providing additional nourishment to compromised skin.

While water-based peptides actively stimulate repair at a cellular level, oil-based peptides primarily support the skin's surface, helping to restore its protective function and resilience against environmental aggressors.

Hydrophilic vs. Lipophilic: Understanding Skin Absorption

The skin is a complex organ with distinct hydrophilic (water-loving) and lipophilic (oil-loving) environments. Understanding this difference is key to appreciating how formulations interact with the skin:

• Hydrophilic molecules (like water-based peptides) are attracted to water and diffuse readily through aqueous pathways, making them effective at penetrating the hydrated layers of the epidermis.

• Lipophilic molecules (like oil-based peptides and lipid-encapsulated actives) are attracted to fats and integrate well into the lipid matrix of the stratum corneum, enhancing their ability to reinforce barrier function.

This duality underpins the concept of strategic layering in post-treatment care: applying hydrophilic actives first to target cellular repair, followed by lipophilic formulations to seal in moisture and protect the newly treated skin.

Application in Aesthetic Practice

For optimal outcomes, practitioners should advise clients to:

1. Begin with water-based peptides immediately post-treatment to capitalize on the skin's heightened permeability.
2. Introduce oil-based peptides 48 hours later to nourish and restore the skin barrier as it begins to re-establish itself.

This two-phase approach leverages the strengths of both hydrophilic and lipophilic peptides, supporting deep cellular repair and surface barrier restoration for truly regenerative results.

Wharton's Jelly: Signaling Cell-Rich Matrix for Skin Rejuvenation

Wharton's Jelly (WJ), often referred to as the "biologic treasure of the umbilical cord," is revolutionizing regenerative aesthetics with its unique ability to stimulate profound skin renewal. As a naturally occurring gelatinous connective tissue found within the umbilical cord, Wharton's Jelly contains an abundance of mesenchymal signaling cells, growth factors, cytokines, and extracellular matrix proteins that are critical for tissue repair and regeneration.

What is Wharton's Jelly?

Wharton's Jelly is the cushioning substance surrounding the umbilical cord's blood vessels. It provides structural support and protects the cord during pregnancy. Rich in mesenchymal signaling cells (MSCs), hyaluronic acid, collagen, and glycosaminoglycans (GAGs), it serves as a biologically active matrix with significant anti-inflammatory and regenerative properties.

When processed for medical and aesthetic use, Wharton's Jelly is purified to remove cells and DNA while preserving its rich reservoir of bioactive molecules. This cell-free preparation ensures safety while retaining regenerative benefits.

Regenerative Components of Wharton's Jelly

The potency of Wharton's Jelly lies in its composition:

• Mesenchymal Signaling Cells (MSCs): Secrete trophic factors that stimulate tissue repair, modulate inflammation, and encourage angiogenesis.
• Growth Factors: Including transforming growth factor-beta (TGF-β), platelet-derived growth factor (PDGF), and vascular endothelial growth factor (VEGF), which drive fibroblast activity and collagen production.

• Hyaluronic Acid: Provides intense hydration and supports extracellular matrix integrity.
• Extracellular Vesicles (EVs): Exosomes and micro vesicles that facilitate intercellular communication and cellular reprogramming.

Aesthetic Applications of Wharton's Jelly

Wharton's Jelly has emerged as a valuable tool in the aesthetic toolbox, particularly for clients seeking advanced regenerative treatments:

• Microneedling with WJ: Applied post-microneedling, Wharton's Jelly penetrates microchannels to deliver its bioactive components directly to the dermal layer, accelerating healing and enhancing collagen remodeling.
• Injectable WJ Treatments (where permitted): Used in some clinical settings to support dermal volume, elasticity, and repair of scar tissue.
• Post-Laser Recovery: Reduces inflammation, speeds re-epithelialization, and minimizes downtime after ablative procedures.
• Anti-Aging Facials: Provide deep hydration, barrier support, and cellular nourishment when used topically in luxury treatments.

Clinical Impact and Future Directions

Early studies and clinical use cases suggest Wharton's Jelly is particularly effective for improving:

*Fine lines and wrinkles

*Skin laxity

*Uneven texture and scarring

*Stretch marks and post-inflammatory pigmentation

As research progresses, Wharton's Jelly is poised to become a cornerstone of regenerative aesthetics, offering a biologically rich alternative to traditional dermal fillers or synthetic growth factor serums.

The Overuse and Misuse of "Stem Cells" in Aesthetics and Regenerative Medicine

In recent years, the term "stem cell" has become a buzzword in both the medical and aesthetic industries. It evokes images of miraculous healing, youthful regeneration, and cutting-edge science. Unfortunately, the popularity of the term has led to widespread misuse and misunderstanding, both by marketing teams eager to capitalize on consumer interest and by practitioners who may not fully grasp the science behind it.

The Stem Cell Buzzword Problem

In aesthetics, the phrase "stem cell therapy" often appears on product labels, treatment menus, and advertisements. However, in most cases:

- No live stem cells are present. Instead, these products contain extracts, growth factors, or conditioned media derived from cultured cells.
- The term is used loosely to describe biologics, such as exosomes, amniotic fluid, or Wharton's Jelly, even though these are cell-free therapies containing signaling molecules rather than living stem cells.
- Consumer expectations are inflated, leading to confusion about what treatments can realistically achieve.

Arnold Caplan was the scientist who originally coined the term Mesenchymal Stem Cells, often referred to as MSCs. Over time, however, his understanding of these cells evolved. Rather than functioning primarily as replacement cells that become new tissue, he recognized that their most important role was communication. In his 2017 paper, *Mesenchymal Stem Cells: Time to Change the Name!* Caplan proposed renaming them Medicinal Signaling Cells to more accurately reflect what they do. These cells send signals that help regulate inflammation, support repair, and guide the body's natural healing processes. This shift in language marked a significant turning point in regenerative medicine and aligns closely with the core idea that healing is not driven by force, but by restoring the signals the body already understands.

The FDA has even issued warnings about unproven "stem cell" therapies, particularly when claims extend beyond the evidence or involve unregulated procedures.

Understanding the Science: What Are Stem Cells?

True stem cells are undifferentiated cells with the remarkable ability to:

1. Self-renew (produce more stem cells)
2. Differentiate into specialized cell types (e.g., skin, muscle, nerve)

They are used in highly controlled environments for research and some medical applications, such as bone marrow transplants.

In aesthetics, however, most therapies marketed as "stem cell" are actually using cellular derivatives: proteins, growth factors, and extracellular vesicles secreted by stem cells during culture. While these biologics are powerful in supporting skin rejuvenation, they are not stem cells themselves.

The Difference: Mesenchymal Signaling Cells vs. Mesenchymal Stem Cells

Feature	Mesenchymal Stem Cells (MSCs)	Mesenchymal Signaling Cells (MSiCs)
Definition	Undifferentiated cells capable of self-renewal and differentiation.	Cells or cell fragments that release regenerative signals but lack stemness.
Function	Can divide and differentiate into bone, cartilage, fat, and connective tissue cells.	Act as messengers to regulate healing and repair via paracrine signaling.
Presence in Aesthetics	Rarely used directly; requires strict laboratory and regulatory control.	Found in biologics like Wharton's Jelly and amniotic fluid in a cell-free form.
Safety	Must be carefully controlled due to risk of unwanted differentiation or immune reaction.	Safer as they contain no living cells—only signaling molecules.

Why This Matters

Understanding this distinction is critical:

- Mesenchymal Stem Cells are living, undifferentiated cells requiring regulatory oversight.

- Mesenchymal Signaling Cells, or more accurately, their secreted factors, provide the therapeutic benefits in many aesthetic biologics without the complexity or risk of stem cell therapy.

This clarity helps practitioners and clients set realistic expectations and fosters a more ethical approach to regenerative aesthetics.

MSC Exosomes VS Purified Amniotic Fluid in Skin Health

As regenerative aesthetics continues to evolve, practitioners are increasingly presented with advanced biologics that promise cellular-level repair and rejuvenation. Two such innovations, Mesenchymal Signaling Cell (MSC) Exosomes and Purified Amniotic Fluid, are often discussed in the same breath. However, while they share regenerative properties, their composition, mechanisms of action, and applications in skin health are distinctly different.

What Are MSC Exosomes?

Exosomes are nano-sized extracellular vesicles released by cells that act as messengers, facilitating communication between cells. When derived from MSCs, now more accurately referred to as mesenchymal signaling cells, these exosomes carry bioactive signals that help guide processes such as repair, inflammation regulation, and regeneration. Rather than functioning as replacement cells, MSCs play a primary role in communication, and their exosomes reflect this by delivering instructions that support the skin and body's natural healing responses.

MSC exosomes are rich in proteins, lipids, microRNAs (miRNAs), and growth factors that play key roles in tissue repair and immune modulation. Their small size allows them to penetrate deeply into the skin, delivering their payload of bioactive molecules directly to target cells.

Key Attributes of MSC Exosomes:

- Act as signaling molecules to activate cellular repair pathways.
- Contain a highly concentrated and purified set of growth factors and cytokines.
- Typically created through laboratory processes isolating exosomes from MSC cultures.
- Favorable for post-procedural recovery (microneedling, lasers) where fast healing and reduced inflammation are desired.

What Is Purified Amniotic Fluid?

Purified amniotic fluid, on the other hand, is a naturally occurring biologic harvested from donated, ethically sourced placental tissue during full-term cesarean sections. Purified amniotic fluid contains a broad orchestra of biologic components, including exosomes (from the amniotic cells), growth factors, cytokines, hyaluronic acid, anti-inflammatory proteins, and unique molecules like Klotho, a protein associated with anti-aging effects.

Key Attributes of Purified Amniotic Fluid:
- Contains a wide variety of growth factors and bioactive molecules.
- Offers anti-inflammatory, antimicrobial, and pro-healing effects.
- Hydrates and nourishes the skin while supporting barrier repair.
- Ideal for post-procedural application and standalone rejuvenation treatments.

Why Choose One Over the Other?

In practice, the choice between MSC exosomes and Purified Amniotic Fluid depends on treatment goals:
- MSC Exosomes excel in highly targeted cellular repair and are ideal for intensive rejuvenation post-aggressive procedures.
- Purified Amniotic Fluid shines in hydrating, soothing, and supporting overall skin recovery due to its broad array of biologics. Practitioners tend to see faster healing results with

PAF rather than just using MSC Exosomes.
Some practitioners even combine both in layered treatment protocols, applying MSC exosomes for deep cellular activation, followed by amniotic fluid to nourish and fortify the skin barrier.

The Synergy of Science and Nature

While MSC exosomes represent a cutting-edge, lab-engineered approach to regenerative skin care, Purified Amniotic Fluid reflects the natural complexity of biologics as found in the human body. Both offer powerful tools for skin professionals seeking to elevate their treatments beyond traditional cosmeceuticals. Understanding their unique properties allows estheticians and medical providers to make informed choices and customize protocols that best serve their clients' needs

Chapter 4

Treatment Pairings and Protocols

Microneedling + Exosomes

Microneedling and exosome therapy represent a powerful combination in regenerative aesthetics. Together, they optimize the skin's healing response, enhance cellular communication, and deliver dramatic improvements in texture, tone, and overall skin quality.

Why Combine Microneedling with Exosomes?

Microneedling involves the controlled creation of micro-injuries in the epidermis and dermis using fine needles. This process initiates the skin's natural wound healing cascade, triggering fibroblast activation and collagen production.

Exosomes, nano-sized extracellular vesicles secreted by stem cells, act as biological messengers. They carry proteins, growth factors, RNA, and lipids that facilitate intercellular communication and promote tissue regeneration.

By applying exosomes immediately post-needling, these bioactive molecules penetrate deeply into the microchannels created by the device. The result:

* Enhanced delivery of regenerative signals

*Accelerated repair of damaged tissue

*Reduction of inflammation and downtime

*Superior improvements in skin texture, elasticity, and pigmentation

Protocol: Microneedling + Exosomes

Treatment Goal: Skin rejuvenation, acne scarring, and pigmentation correction

Pre-Treatment Preparation

Obtain informed consent and review contraindications.

- Cleanse skin thoroughly with a gentle, pH-balanced cleanser.
- Degrease the skin with a prep solution (Hypochlorous Acid) to ensure sterility.
- Apply topical anesthetic (5–7% lidocaine cream) for 20–30 minutes; remove completely before starting.

Cleanse skin again after removing the anesthetic

Microneedling Procedure

- Use a professional-grade microneedling device with sterile, single-use needle cartridges.

Use Hyaluronic Acid as your glide

• Set depth according to treatment area:

- 0.25–0.5 mm for thin skin (forehead, periorbital)
- 0.75–1.5 mm for thicker skin (cheeks, jawline)
- 1.5–2.0 mm for scars (supervised by medical provider if applicable)

• Perform uniform passes in horizontal, vertical, and diagonal directions until mild erythema and pinpoint bleeding are observed.

Exosome Application

• Immediately post-needling, apply 1–2 ml of purified exosome solution evenly to the treated area.

• Gently massage to facilitate absorption through microchannels.

• Optionally, apply a hydrating, sterile sheet mask (e.g., cellulose mask) to soothe and lock in moisture.

Post-Treatment Care

• Advise the client to avoid makeup, heat exposure, and active skincare ingredients (retinoids, AHAs) for 72 hours.

• Provide a gentle cleanser and moisturizer for home use.

• Encourage daily broad-spectrum SPF 30+ to protect healing skin.

Treatment Schedule

Recommend a series of 3–6 treatments spaced 4–6 weeks apart for optimal results. Maintenance treatments every 6–12 months can sustain improvements.

Clinical Insights

• Studies show that combining exosomes with microneedling reduces downtime by 20–30% and improves collagen deposition compared to microneedling alone.

• Ideal for clients with sensitive or compromised skin due to the anti-inflammatory properties of exosomes.

Dermaplaning + Purified Amniotic Fluid

Dermaplaning and the application of purified amniotic fluid form a synergistic combination for advanced skin rejuvenation. This pairing not only enhances treatment efficacy but also promotes a faster recovery and a more luminous, hydrated complexion.

Why Combine Dermaplaning with Purified Amniotic Fluid?

Dermaplaning is a physical exfoliation method that removes the stratum corneum—the outermost layer of dead skin cells and fine vellus hair (peach fuzz). This process creates an ultra-smooth surface, primes the skin for maximal absorption of active ingredients, and encourages cell turnover.

Purified amniotic fluid, derived from ethically sourced and donated placental tissue, contains a rich blend of growth factors, cytokines, proteins, and hyaluronic acid. When applied immediately after dermaplaning, these biologic components penetrate more effectively and support:
*Anti-inflammatory action to calm post-treatment redness
*Hydration replenishment and skin barrier repair
*Acceleration of cellular repair and collagen synthesis

Protocol: Dermaplaning + Purified Amniotic Fluid

Treatment Goal: Instant glow, improved hydration, enhanced recovery post-procedure

Pre-Treatment Preparation

• Obtain informed consent and review contraindications (e.g., active acne, open lesions).
• Cleanse skin thoroughly with a gentle, pH-balanced cleanser to remove makeup and impurities.
• Degrease skin with Velez HOCL (Hypochlorous Acid) solution to allow smooth blade movement.

Dermaplaning Procedure

• Use a sterile, single-use surgical blade (e.g., #10 blade) on dry skin.

• Hold skin taut and gently scrape at a 45-degree angle using feather-light strokes.

• Work systematically across the face, avoiding areas of active breakouts or irritation.

• Remove any loosened debris with a soft, dry gauze.

Purified Amniotic Fluid Application

• Apply 1–2 ml of purified amniotic fluid evenly across the freshly derma planed skin.

• Use gloved hands to gently press and massage the fluid to aid absorption.

• Optionally, apply a chilled cellulose sheet mask to soothe the skin and enhance penetration.

Post-Treatment Care

• Apply a calming serum or moisturizer suitable for post-procedure skin.

• Advise the client to avoid sun exposure and active skincare (retinoids, acids) for 72 hours.

• Encourage daily use of a mineral SPF 30+ to protect the rejuvenated skin.

Treatment Schedule

This combination is ideal as a stand-alone monthly treatment or as a pre-treatment protocol before more intensive procedures (e.g., chemical peels, RF microneedling).

Clinical Insights

- Clients often report reduced redness and irritation compared to dermaplaning alone.
- Excellent option for clients with sensitive or compromised skin who may not tolerate more aggressive treatments.
- Can be offered as part of a deluxe "Red Carpet Glow" facial service.

LED Therapy + Peptides and LED Therapy + PAF

LED (Light Emitting Diode) therapy has emerged as a cornerstone of non-invasive skin rejuvenation. Using specific wavelengths of light, LED devices stimulate photo-biomodulation, a process where light energy penetrates the skin and triggers cellular responses. When combined with bioactive topicals such as peptides or amniotic fluid, the synergy between light and biologics leads to enhanced absorption, improved skin repair, and faster results.

Why Combine LED Therapy with Biologics?

LED light, particularly in the red (630–660 nm) and near-infrared (800–880 nm) spectra, penetrates the dermis and stimulates mitochondrial activity, increasing ATP production. This surge in cellular energy supports:

1. Collagen and elastin synthesis
2. Enhanced circulation and lymphatic drainage
3. Reduced inflammation and redness
4. Accelerated wound healing

What Does Increasing ATP Production Mean?

ATP (adenosine triphosphate) is the primary energy currency of the cell, produced in the mitochondria. When LED therapy stimulates mitochondrial activity, it enhances the production of ATP. This increase in cellular energy allows skin cells, especially fibroblasts and keratinocytes, to function more efficiently. They can repair damage, synthesize new collagen and elastin fibers, and regenerate tissue at a faster rate. In simple terms, more ATP means the skin has more energy to heal, renew, and rejuvenate.

Protocol 1: LED Therapy + Peptides

Treatment Goal: Improve skin firmness, elasticity, and hydration while reducing fine lines.

Pre-Treatment Preparation

- Cleanse skin with a gentle, non-irritating cleanser.
- Lightly exfoliate if needed to remove surface debris and enhance product penetration.

LED Therapy

- Use an FDA-cleared LED device with red and near-infrared wavelengths.
- Session Duration: 20–30 minutes, depending on device specifications.
- Position the device 1–2 inches above the treatment area, ensuring even light distribution.

Peptide Serum Application

- Immediately after LED therapy, apply a peptide-rich serum (containing copper peptides, growth factor peptides, or signal peptides).
- Gently massage to ensure even coverage.
- End with a cooling sheet mask for added hydration and penetration.

Post-Treatment Care

- Apply a barrier-repair moisturizer to lock in peptides.
- Recommend broad-spectrum SPF 30+ for daily use.

Protocol 2: LED Therapy + PAF

Treatment Goal: Accelerate healing, reduce redness, and rejuvenate stressed or compromised skin.

Pre-Treatment Preparation

- Cleanse and prepare skin as above.
- Assess for contraindications (active infections, photosensitivity disorders).

LED Therapy

- Use red and/or near-infrared light for anti-inflammatory and regenerative effects.
- Session Duration: 20–30 minutes.

Purified Amniotic Fluid Application

- Apply 1–2 ml of purified amniotic fluid immediately post-LED session.
- Massage gently for optimal absorption.
- Follow with a chilled, sterile cellulose mask and leave on for 20 minutes.

Post-Treatment Care

- Apply a calming moisturizer or serum.
- Advise clients to avoid heat exposure and active skincare ingredients for 72 hours.

Clinical Insights

- Pairing LED therapy with peptides is ideal for clients seeking anti-aging benefits and enhanced skin firmness.
- Combining LED therapy with amniotic fluid is excellent for post-procedure recovery, sensitive skin, and inflammatory conditions such as rosacea.
- Both protocols can be performed weekly or bi-weekly as part of a rejuvenation series.

Post-Treatment Care and Absorption Optimization

Proper post-treatment care is the cornerstone of achieving optimal results with biologic-based therapies. While biologics such as exosomes, peptides, and amniotic fluid provide powerful regenerative signals, their efficacy can be significantly enhanced or diminished based on how the skin is cared for in the critical hours and days following treatment.

Why Post-Treatment Care Matters

After treatments like microneedling, LED therapy, or dermaplaning, the skin's barrier function is temporarily compromised. Microchannels created during these procedures allow for deeper penetration of active ingredients, but they also increase vulnerability to irritation, dehydration, and environmental stressors. Proper aftercare supports:

1. Enhanced absorption of biologics for deeper cellular repair
2. Reduced inflammation and faster recovery
3. Prevention of complications such as post-inflammatory hyperpigmentation (PIH) or infection

Key Post-Treatment Guidelines

Avoid:

- Harsh products: Retinoids, alpha hydroxy acids (AHAs), beta hydroxy acids (BHAs), and physical exfoliants for 5-7 days.
- Heat exposure: Saunas, steam rooms, hot yoga, and intense exercise for 72 hours.
- Direct sun exposure: UV rays can exacerbate irritation and delay healing. Avoid for 72 hours

Recommended:

- Gentle Cleansing: Use a mild, pH-balanced cleanser twice daily.

• Barrier Repair: After 48 hours, you will want to begin to support the barrier in its repair process by using a rich fat-soluble oil and moisturizer.

• Hydration Support: Hyaluronic acid-based serums help maintain moisture levels and support biologic ingredient absorption. Using a water-based serum in the first 48 hours is essential.

• Sun Protection: Broad-spectrum SPF 30+ daily to prevent photo-damage and pigmentary changes.

Supporting Biologic Absorption

To maximize the activity of biologics post-treatment, consider:

• Recovery Masks: Apply a chilled hydrogel or cellulose mask to calm skin and enhance penetration.

• Layering Protocols: Use biologic serums first (to allow direct absorption), followed by occlusive moisturizers to seal them in.

• Avoid Occlusives Too Soon: Wait 12–24 hours post-procedure before applying thick occlusive balms unless directed, as they may trap heat and prolong redness. Also, pay attention to ingredients so they don't counteract the choice of biologic used on the skin. Amniotic and Warton's Jelly are sensitive to preservatives and alcohol in skincare.

Clinical Pearl of Wisdom

Encourage clients to commit to a home care routine tailored to their treatment type. Consistency in hydration and barrier repair amplifies the regenerative potential of in-office biologic treatments. A monthly treatment in the office is maintained by a good home care routine.

Chapter 5

Safety, Ethics, and Scope

Legal Considerations and Working with a Medical Director

As the aesthetic industry continues to embrace advanced treatments and biologics, estheticians and spa professionals must operate within their legal scope of practice. Understanding the regulations that govern aesthetic procedures not only protects the client but also safeguards the practitioner's license and reputation.

The Role of the Medical Director

For estheticians seeking to integrate biologics or medical-grade treatments into their practice, collaborating with a medical director is essential. A medical director provides the necessary supervision and delegation required for procedures outside of the esthetician's scope.

Benefits of Working with a Medical Director:

- Ensures compliance with state and federal regulations.
- Allows access to advanced treatments like PRP, Purified

Amniotic Fluid, and Wharton's Jelly under appropriate oversight.

• Supports professional development through training and protocol development.

• Enhances credibility and patient trust by demonstrating medical partnership.

There are a few companies out there that will provide you with a medical director for a setup fee and a monthly fee. We Treat is a company with medical directors ready to cover in all 50 states.

Delegation vs. Direct Supervision

It is important to understand the difference between delegation and supervision:

• Delegation: The medical director assigns specific tasks to qualified staff but remains ultimately responsible.

• Direct Supervision: The medical director must be physically present on-site during the procedure (required in some states for certain advanced treatments).

State boards and medical boards dictate these requirements. Always verify what level of oversight is required for your specific treatments.

Ensuring Legal Compliance

To stay compliant:

1. Consult State Board Regulations: Review the esthetician scope of practice and licensing laws for your state.
2. Obtain Proper Training: Complete advanced certifications approved by your state board before offering higher-level procedures.
3. Establish Written Protocols: Work with your medical director to create clear, signed protocols for all advanced services.
4. Maintain Detailed Records: Document every treatment, consent form, and delegation agreement.

Key Takeaway

While biologics and advanced aesthetic treatments offer exciting growth opportunities, they require careful navigation of the legal landscape. Partnering with a qualified medical director ensures safe, ethical, and compliant practice, allowing estheticians to expand their services without overstepping professional boundaries.

Storage and Handling of Biologic Materials

The use of biologics in aesthetic practice, such as exosomes, purified amniotic fluid, Wharton's Jelly, and other cellular derivatives, requires strict attention to storage and handling protocols. These advanced therapeutics are sensitive to environmental conditions, and improper management can compromise their efficacy and safety.

Storage: Preserving Potency

Biologic materials are inherently delicate. Their bioactive components—growth factors, cytokines, extracellular vesicles, and peptides—can degrade when exposed to heat, light, or moisture. To maintain potency:

- Follow Manufacturer Instructions: Each product comes with specific storage guidelines (e.g., –20°C or –80°C for cryopreserved biologics). If you order a product that has live cell components, you will need a -150 ultra-low freezer for storage. Many manufacturers have validated shipping for 48 hours, so you can plan your treatments for shipping arrival and go without freezers.
- Freezer Requirements: Store biologics in medical-grade freezers with temperature monitoring systems to avoid fluctuations.
- Light Protection: Keep products in original packaging or opaque containers to prevent photodegradation.
- Avoid Freeze-Thaw Cycles: Repeated freezing and thawing

can damage proteins and vesicles. Only thaw immediately before use and discard any unused portion.

Handling: Maintaining Sterility

Sterility is paramount when working with biologic materials to prevent contamination that could lead to infection or inflammatory reactions.

- Use Aseptic Technique: Always handle biologics in a clean environment using gloves, sterile instruments, and, if possible, a laminar flow hood for preparation.
- Single-Use Policy: Most biologic products are intended for single-use only and should never be re-entered or stored once opened. Re-freezing a biologic will ruin the product.
- Reconstitution Protocols: For lyophilized (freeze-dried) biologics, use sterile saline or other approved diluents as directed. Mix gently to avoid denaturing sensitive components.

Quality Control and Regulatory Compliance

Proper documentation ensures traceability and compliance with regulatory requirements:

- Track Lot Numbers and Expiration Dates: Record every product's lot number and expiry date in client files.

• Chain of Custody: Document receipt, storage conditions, and use to ensure a clear chain of custody for each biologic.
• Disposal of Expired Materials: Follow biohazard protocols for disposal of expired or unused biologic products.

Incorrect storage or handling can render biologics inactive, leading to poor clinical outcomes and potential liability for the practitioner. By adhering to strict protocols, aesthetic professionals uphold patient safety, product integrity, and professional standards.

Consent Forms and Client Education

In the realm of aesthetic medicine and regenerative treatments, obtaining informed consent is not just a regulatory requirement; it is the foundation of ethical and professional practice. Biologic-based therapies such as exosomes, purified amniotic fluid, and Wharton's Jelly require special attention to client understanding due to their advanced nature and emerging science.

The Importance of Informed Consent

Informed consent is a legal and ethical process in which clients are educated about the treatment they are about to receive. It ensures that:

- The client understands the procedure, including what it involves and how it works.
- Potential risks, side effects, and contraindications are clearly explained.
- Alternative treatments are discussed when applicable.
- The client has the opportunity to ask questions and make an informed decision.

For biologic-based services, this process is especially critical because clients may have preconceived notions about "stem cells" or "growth factors" that need clarification.

It is also important to note that most manufacturers of biologics do not provide consent forms as part of their product packaging or protocols. This responsibility falls to the practitioner to create and use proper consent documentation.

Educating the Client

Client education begins well before the treatment and should continue throughout the client relationship. Best practices include:

• Pre-Treatment Consultation: Explain the science behind the biologic being used, how it supports skin repair, and what results to realistically expect.

• Printed Materials: Provide brochures or handouts that outline the treatment, post-care instructions, and possible outcomes.

• Transparency About Evidence: Discuss the current research supporting biologic use in aesthetics while noting that outcomes may vary.

• Visual Aids: Use before-and-after photos, diagrams, or videos to help clients visualize the process and results.

Documenting Consent

Every biologic treatment should be accompanied by a signed consent form that includes:

• The name of the biologic product and its manufacturer.

• A description of how the product will be applied or administered.

• A list of potential risks and complications (e.g., redness, swelling, allergic reaction).

• Acknowledgment of off-label use (if applicable).

• Confirmation that post-treatment care instructions were provided and explained.

Maintain these records securely as part of the client's file for both legal protection and quality assurance.

Failure to obtain proper consent exposes the practitioner to legal risks and can undermine client trust. Conversely, a robust consent and education process empowers clients, sets appropriate expectations, and strengthens the professional relationship.

Sample Biologic Treatment Consent Form

Client Name: ______________________________

Date of Birth: ______________________________

Treatment Date: ____________________________

Practitioner: ______________________________

I hereby consent to receive treatment involving the use of biologic materials, which may include exosomes, purified amniotic fluid, Wharton's Jelly, or other cellular derivatives. I understand that these materials are derived from donated and processed human tissue and are intended to support skin regeneration and healing.

I acknowledge the following:

• The procedure and its purpose have been explained to me in detail.

• I understand the potential risks, including but not limited to redness, swelling, irritation, infection, allergic reaction, or lack of expected results.

• I understand that the use of biologics in aesthetics may be considered off-label and results may vary.

• I have had the opportunity to ask questions and all my concerns have been addressed.

• I understand the post-treatment care instructions and agree to follow them as directed.

Signature of Client: ______________ Date: _________

Signature of Practitioner: ____________Date: _________

Risk Factors and Contraindications

When incorporating biologic-based treatments into a topical aesthetic practice, client safety must always remain the top priority. These advanced therapies, while generally well-tolerated, are not suitable for every individual. A thorough understanding of contraindications and risk factors helps practitioners make informed decisions and avoid adverse outcomes.

Pre-Treatment Screening: (A critical step for any treatment as an Esthetician)

Before initiating any biologic therapy, perform a comprehensive client consultation and medical history review. Key areas to assess include:

- Pregnancy and Breastfeeding: Biologics are not recommended due to limited research on safety in these populations.
- Autoimmune Disorders: Clients with active autoimmune conditions (e.g., lupus, rheumatoid arthritis) may experience unpredictable responses due to altered immune regulation.
- Active Infections: Any bacterial, viral, or fungal infection at the treatment site should be resolved before proceeding.
- Recent Use of Isotretinoin (Accutane): Wait at least 6–12 months after isotretinoin use to minimize risk of skin irritation or poor wound healing.
- Allergies or Sensitivities: Although rare, biologics derived from human tissue may carry a risk of hypersensitivity. Screen for known allergies and consider patch testing when appropriate.

Potential Adverse Reactions

Even with appropriate screening, practitioners should be aware of possible complications and be prepared to manage them:

- Localized Reactions: Redness, swelling, bruising, or discomfort at the application site.
- Delayed Hypersensitivity: Rare cases of inflammatory responses days after treatment.
- Infection: A small risk if aseptic techniques are not strictly followed.
- Ineffectiveness: Variability in client response based on age, health status, or underlying conditions.

Emergency Preparedness

Practices offering biologic treatments should have protocols in place for managing adverse events, including:

- Access to antihistamines and epinephrine for allergic reactions.
- Clear referral pathways to medical providers for unexpected complications.
- Staff training in recognizing and responding to adverse events.

When to Refer

Always err on the side of caution. If a client presents with a complex medical history, active dermatological conditions, or is otherwise outside the practitioner's scope of expertise, refer them to a licensed medical provider for evaluation.

Contraindications Checklist for Treatment Rooms

_____Pregnancy or breastfeeding

_____Active autoimmune conditions (e.g., lupus, rheumatoid arthritis)

_____Active infection at or near the treatment site

_____History of severe allergic reactions or known hypersensitivity to human tissue-derived products

_____Recent isotretinoin (Accutane) use within the past 6–12 months

_____Poor wound healing or history of keloid formation

_____Uncontrolled diabetes or vascular conditions

_____Current chemotherapy or immunosuppressive therapy

_____ Any other medical condition requiring physician clearance before advanced aesthetic treatment

When it comes to consent, risks, and complications, you want to refer to your liability providers and make sure you are using the proper forms. Everything provided here is for reference only, to give you a place for thought and the process of understanding.

Chapter 6

Clinical Application & Case Studies

Biologics have become a cornerstone in regenerative aesthetics due to their ability to promote natural healing, stimulate collagen production, and enhance skin rejuvenation. This section provides expanded information with clinical evidence, real-world case examples, and integration protocols for aesthetic practice.

Clinical Studies Supporting Biologic Use

• **Microneedling with PRP for Acne Scars:**

A systematic review of 14 studies showed that microneedling combined with PRP provides significantly better outcomes for acne scar improvement compared to microneedling alone. Patients reported faster healing and improved scar texture.

(Reference: Frontiers in Medicine, 2021)

• **Exosomes in Skin Rejuvenation:**

Clinical data demonstrate that topical exosomes applied post-microneedling reduce pigmentation and inflammation,

while promoting even skin tone and texture without post-inflammatory hyperpigmentation.
(Reference: MDPI Applied Sciences, 2023)

• **Wharton's Jelly for Advanced Healing:**
Emerging studies on Wharton's Jelly-derived mesenchymal signaling cells show enhanced dermal repair and faster recovery in patients undergoing aesthetic treatments, supporting its use in post-laser and post-microneedling recovery.

Real-World Case Examples

Case 1: Acne Scar Revision with PRP
A 30-year-old female with moderate atrophic acne scars underwent a series of six microneedling sessions combined with PRP every 4 weeks. Post-treatment, the patient experienced a 45% improvement in scar depth and overall skin smoothness. Side effects were limited to mild erythema resolving within 48 hours.

Case 2: Facial Rejuvenation with Exosomes
In a clinical setting, exosomes were applied topically post-RF microneedling in a 45-year-old patient presenting with fine lines and mild laxity. The patient reported visible

improvement in skin firmness and radiance within 3 weeks, with reduced redness and downtime.

Integration Protocols and Dosing Guidelines

• **Microneedling + Biologics:** Apply 2–3 mL of PRP, PAF, or exosomes immediately post-microneedling at 0.25–0.5 mm depth.

• **Post-Laser Recovery:** Topically apply biologics as a serum for 5–7 days post-procedure to reduce inflammation and accelerate healing.

Client-Facing Post-Care Summary

After receiving biologic-enhanced treatments, patients should avoid sun exposure, use gentle cleansers, and apply SPF daily. Redness and mild swelling may occur but usually subside within 24–48 hours.

References

1. Frontiers in Medicine (2021). Microneedling with PRP in Acne Scar Management.
2. MDPI Applied Sciences (2023). The Use of Exosomes in Aesthetic Skin Treatments.
3. ClinicalTrials.gov (Ongoing). Regenerative Potential of Wharton's Jelly-derived Products.

4. Vogue & Allure Features (2023). Real-World Experiences with Exosome Therapy.

Chapter 7

Closing Reflections

The Future of Biologics and My Practice Philosophy

As I bring this book to a close, I feel a deep sense of gratitude and responsibility. Gratitude for the science that has given us access to powerful biologics like Purified Amniotic Fluid and Wharton's Jelly, and responsibility to share what I've learned in a way that empowers estheticians, medical professionals, and anyone passionate about skin health.

My gratitude to Dr. Ian White for his kindness and for having the ability to work with him over the past few years. His wisdom is beyond words. I am forever grateful to learn from him and walk with him in the field of regenerative science. Dr Ian White is the CEO and CSO of Neobiosis, and my friend.

Over the years, my work has taught me a simple truth: the skin already knows how to heal itself. It is brilliantly designed to repair, renew, and protect. Our role as professionals is not to force change, but to provide the right tools and the right "food", so the skin can do what it's programmed to do.

This philosophy has shaped how I approach every treatment. I've moved away from harsh, aggressive interventions and toward therapies that support and amplify the skin's innate wisdom. Biologics have been the key to unlocking this gentle yet profoundly effective approach.

Why Purified Amniotic Fluid Holds a Special Place

Among the biologics I've worked with, Purified Amniotic Fluid stands out as a favorite. It's often described as the full orchestra, and I couldn't agree more. Unlike isolated molecules or single growth factors, Purified Amniotic Fluid delivers a symphony of ingredients: exosomes, growth factors, cytokines, hyaluronic acid, and rare proteins like Klotho. Together, these elements create a balanced and harmonious environment for skin regeneration.

I've seen the results firsthand in my treatment room. Post-microneedling, clients experience less redness and irritation. Their skin heals faster, with a noticeable glow and improved texture. Scars soften, fine lines diminish, and hydration is restored. There's a holistic quality to the transformation, one that feels aligned with the skin's natural processes rather than imposed upon them.

My Recommended Products for Skin Professionals

To support practitioners and clients in maximizing their biologic-based treatments, I recommend incorporating the following into your protocols and home care regimens:

Velez Cellulose Mask – A calming and hydrating post-treatment mask that enhances absorption of biologics like amniotic fluid and exosomes. Its cooling effect soothes the skin and reduces post-procedure inflammation.

Pavise Daily Defense SPF – Sun protection is non-negotiable in regenerative aesthetics. Pavise Daily Defense offers broad-spectrum protection with an elegant, wearable formula that supports barrier repair and protects the investment in biologic treatments.

Lilium® by Neobiosis® - Elevating aesthetic outcomes by harnessing the true origin of beauty. Lilium Pure and Lilium Gelee Pure (purified amniotic fluid and Warton's Jelly Topical Biologic Cosmetics) – www.liliumpure.com

The Future: Topical Wharton's Jelly and Beyond

As we look ahead, the field of regenerative aesthetics is only getting more exciting. One of the most promising frontiers is the development of topical formulations incorporating Wharton's Jelly. This gelatinous substance from umbilical cord tissue is rich in mesenchymal signaling cells, growth factors, and extracellular matrix proteins. Early studies suggest its potential in supporting dermal remodeling, increasing elasticity, and enhancing skin texture.

While current applications of Wharton's Jelly are primarily injectable, researchers are exploring ways to harness its regenerative power in topical formats that could become game-changers for post-procedural care and anti-aging treatments.

Other emerging discoveries include nano-encapsulation of biologics for improved penetration and the combination of biologics with advanced delivery systems like LED therapy, ultrasound, and transdermal patches. The future is bright, and I am thrilled to see how these innovations will continue to elevate what we can offer our clients.

My Closing Message to You

When I started writing, I hoped to put together something that could serve as a helpful resource, a combination of glossary, guide, and sample protocols to offer a place to begin as we navigate the world of biologics together. It's not meant to be definitive or all-encompassing, but rather a starting point for curiosity and creativity in our work.

This area of aesthetics is rapidly evolving, and with that growth comes both innovation and misinformation. While there is still much to learn, the goal of this book is to provide a thoughtful, science-informed foundation built from education, clinical experience, collaboration, and ongoing exploration within regenerative aesthetics.

Through years of hands-on practice, research, and partnership with professionals in the regenerative medicine space, I have seen the growing potential of biologic ingredients to support skin health, recovery, and advanced aesthetic treatments. I hope this information helps practitioners better understand these technologies, approach them responsibly, and integrate them with confidence, professionalism, and respect for the skin's natural processes.

Think of this as an invitation to keep exploring. Use what resonates, leave what doesn't, and let it inspire your own journey in this evolving space. We all have so much to learn, but I believe that together we can continue growing, one client and one treatment at a time.

Remember, the doctors need us as partners. We bring a unique perspective to the table, one grounded in touch, observation, and a deep understanding of the skin's rhythms.

Most importantly, never lose the joy in what you do. This is a beautiful field filled with opportunities to change lives, one face at a time. Continue to explore, innovate, and believe in the extraordinary healing power of the skin.

Because when we work with the skin; not against it, we create results that are not only transformative but also sustainable.

About the Author

Amy Jo Roberts, LE, is a licensed esthetician, regenerative aesthetics educator, author, and Founder of The Veil™ educational platform. With more than a decade of hands-on clinical esthetics experience across multiple states and over 25 years in business development, sales, and executive leadership, Amy has become recognized for her ability to bridge aesthetic science, skin communication, and the evolving world of regenerative skincare education.

Her work is rooted in helping professionals better understand how the skin communicates through symptoms, barrier function, inflammation, and recovery. Known for translating complex biologic and regenerative concepts into clear, practical education, Amy has developed advanced training programs focused on biologics, consultation strategy, treatment coordination, post-care optimization, and professional treatment integration.

Amy is the author of *Biologics and Skin Health*, as well as additional educational works centered around regenerative aesthetics, skin behavior, and The Veil™ philosophy. Her teaching emphasizes working with the skin rather than against it, focusing on timing, readiness, coordination, and supporting the skin's natural processes instead of overwhelming it.

Through The Veil™ online education platform, Amy offers advanced professional courses designed for estheticians, medical professionals, and skin health practitioners seeking a deeper understanding of biologics and modern regenerative aesthetics. The *Biologics and Skin Health* course expands on the concepts introduced in her book by providing more in-depth education surrounding biologically active ingredients, skin communication, treatment pairing, barrier support, consultation methodology, post-treatment care, and ethical treatment integration within professional aesthetic practice.

Her educational approach combines science-backed concepts with real-world clinical perspective, helping practitioners gain greater clarity, confidence, and strategy in how they approach advanced skincare and regenerative technologies.

To learn more about online courses, advanced education, and The Veil™ training opportunities, visit: www.theveilgroup.com Use Code: **BIOLOGICS** for our Biologics and Skin Health Course and receive a discount for purchasing this book.